Nutrition Made E-Z

Copyright © 2013

Revised 2020 by A.J. Fleming, N.D.

www.healselfnaturally.weebly.com[1]

DEDICATION

To God, Our Creator, The Greatest Healer
Of Them All.

Table of Contents

DISCLAIMER

This book is not intended to prescribe or diagnose illness. Consult your physician for all medical problems. Testing for food allergies is suggested if suspicions arise. Never take high doses of vitamins, minerals, or herbs without medical supervision. Do not begin an exercise program or halt prescribed medications without doctor guidance. For questions about topics presented in this text contact your physician.

INTRODUCTION

Health care and skyrocketing medical costs in the U.S. has reached an all-time crisis. America is the richest nation in the world but also boasts the highest rates of cancer, heart disease, and obesity. Far too many adults and children alike are grossly overweight.

• • • •

Many of this nation's health woes are caused by a deluge of popular and readily available foods that are overloaded with fat, sugar, and salt while simultaneously lacking in essential nutrients such as vitamins, minerals, antioxidants, phytonutrients and fiber. Additionally, a sedentary lifestyle from our obsession with electronics like computers, cable and satellite television, and video games escalates the obesity problem.

• • • •

In this book you will learn how to convert favorite junk foods into healthy meals, plus all you need to know about the basics of eating right for optimum health. If you are confused about nutrition this book offers quick facts at a glance, information on nutrients, healthy foods, do's and don'ts, fitness tips and more. It is designed to offer helpful hints that can prevent ills, shed pounds, make you look better, feel better, and live a longer, healthier & happier life!

• • • •

Designed for simple study. Learn the general basics of nutrition in a weekend. Includes vegetarian-friendly eating tips, herbal medicine and biblical health passages (medicine for your soul). Educational joy for the entire family. Intended for ages 9 to 99.

• • • •

Hopefully, this book will make a difference and help educate people on the fundamentals of a fit lifestyle, and better eating habits for improved health. Good luck and may God bless all those who seek better health, -The Author

ADAPTING TO HEALTHIER FOODS

In order to get our eating habits under control we must change our perceptions about food. Advertisements attempt to propagandize the masses into thinking that food is intended for social fun and entertainment. We often forget that food is designed by God our Creator to be nourishment for the human body.

· · · ·

Americans are not born craving burgers and fries any more than Italians were born craving pasta or Asians were born craving rice. We crave these foods because we were raised on them from an early age. Thus, they became a habit.

· · · ·

Our taste buds have become spoiled rotten to the point where we seldom care for anything that is not loaded with fat, sugar or salt. It's crucial that we overcome our "pampered" taste barriers in order to be successful in rebuilding health.

· · · ·

The more fat, sugar, and salt that you eat, the more you will want. By making healthier substitutions our taste buds and the digestive system will eventually adapt. Soon you will find yourself with cravings for healthy choices instead.

· · · ·

Taste buds can be re-programmed just like a computer. It is entirely possible to change habits and taste buds. Over a period of time, you can discover that many simple and natural foods, such as vegetables, have marvelous flavors all their own. Many basic food staples do not require being buried in tons of fattening butter or rich creamy dressing in order to offer appealing taste. These discoveries will come with the passage of time.

· · · ·

Rome wasn't built in a day, and patience is a virtue, but many people have been known to entirely rejuvenate their health in a time period of ninety days or less. It all depends on you, and remember that your attitude in life determines your altitude.

PREVENTION PAYS

• • • •

Did you know that three out of four illnesses are self-inflicted by poor lifestyle choices? That's an amazing 75%!

- Smoking, abusing drugs or alcohol, and lack of sleep are common hazards which are known to contribute to health problems.
- A lifestyle that embraces proper diet and regular exercise can reduce the risk of many common ills.
- Ailments that are potentially preventable include cancers, heart disease, diabetes, osteoporosis, migraines, arthritis, hemorrhoids, acne, and even Alzheimer's disease.

• • • •

TERRIFIC TRIO
Three main keys to eating right

- Choose a plant-based diet that emphasizes whole fruit, dark-colored vegetables, whole grains and legumes (beans) above all other foods.
- Select lean meats and low-fat dairy items to help manage cholesterol.
- Include fats, sugars, and salt sparingly in your diet.

• • • •

SMART SHOPPER
Have a strategy when entering a grocery store.

- Never shop when hungry.
- Make a list, then stick to it.
- Use a calculator if on a budget.
- Fill your cart with healthy foods first. In particular, focus on the produce department which features whole fruits and vegetables.

- Avoid your weakest areas of temptation (like the soda, snack and pastry isles).
- Prior to checking out, ensure the healthy choices outnumber the less healthy.

. . . .

LABEL LINGO

Are you a label reader? Doing so can work wonders for your health!

- Nutrition labels help consumers avoid excess amounts of fat, cholesterol, calories, sugar, sodium, and chemical preservatives or food additives.
- Food ingredients are listed in order, from the highest amounts down to the lowest.
- Compare labels of similar food products in order to make the smartest selection.

. . . .

BATTLE OF THE BULGE

Obesity can shorten a life span and increase the risk of various ills such as diabetes, heart disease, and certain cancers.

- Want safe and effective weight loss? Simply reduce your total daily calorie intake and increase physical activity. That means moving more and sitting less!
- Avoid weight-reducing fads and gimmicks that don't incorporate balanced nutrition or plans that neglect exercise.

. . . .

FABULOUSLY FIT

Exercise optimizes health and burns calories. Any type of movement is better than none at all.

- Talk to your doctor before starting a fitness plan, and always loosen up first to avoid strained muscles.

- Begin slowly, then increase as your fitness level improves. Aim for 20-40 minutes daily, 3-5 days weekly.
- Walking is highly endorsed for all ages. Simple to perform, it requires no fees or special gear. A daily walk around the block can work wonders.
- Also consider elastic resistance bands, dumbbell weights, yoga, dancing, or any other physical activity that gets you moving more and sitting less.

• • • •

DIVINE DINING
Waistline tips for dining out:

- Scan menus for calorie-conscious options, or ask your server.
- Focus more on salads and fewer appetizers and desserts. Look for restaurants that feature salad bars, but go light on high-fat dressings.
- Avoid overeating by taking half your meal home. Sharing a meal with a friend means half the calories.
- Or, order a child's portion. It's usually smaller.

• • • •

HEALTHY HEARTS
Heart disease is a leading cause of death in the United States.

- Manage cholesterol with a diet low in saturated fats and rich in fiber.
- Exercise elevates the good form of cholesterol (HDL).
- Strive to maintain normal weight.
- Manage stress, limit intake of alcohol, and don't smoke.

• • • •

DASTARDLY DIABETES
Persons who are overweight tend to be more prone to this disease.

- Avoid sugars, refined white flour, excess salt and alcohol.
- Fiber has a controlling effect on blood sugar levels and is naturally

found in wholesome plant foods which include whole grains, legumes (beans), fruits, vegetables, nuts, and seeds.

- Include regular physical activity in your lifestyle based on your doctor's suggestions.

· · · ·

COMBATING CANCER

Believe it or not, research has shown that many types of cancer are actually preventable. To help reduce your risks of becoming a victim:

- Reduce consumption of fatty foods like red meat (beef and pork) and whole dairy products. Opt for low-fat versions instead.
- Various fruits and vegetables contain nutrients that are known to help bolster the body against many cancers, so be sure to eat a wide variety on a regular basis.
- Avoid smoking, excess alcohol consumption, lack of exercise, and chemical food preservatives or food additives whenever possible.
- Learn to manage stress, in terms of not letting it get out of control.

· · · ·

REFRESHING REFRIGERATOR

How you stock your refrigerator is often a reflection on your overall health:

- Fresh vegetables and fruits should outnumber the sugary snacks.
- Meats should be lean, dairy items should be low-fat, and breads should be of the whole grain variety.

· · · ·

PLENTIFUL PANTRY

Sugary treats, sodas, and high-fat snack chips should be scarce.

- Stock wholesome canned goods such as tuna, sardines, beans, nuts, vegetables, and fruits.
- Boxed or packages selections should include whole grains such as high-fiber cereal, whole wheat noodles, multi-grain crackers, and

brown rice.

- Read labels to avoid preservatives, large amounts of fat, sugar and salt.

. . . .

CANTANKEROUS CHOLESTEROL

There are two types of cholesterol; LDL (low-density lipoprotein or the bad cholesterol) and HDL (high-density lipoprotein or the good cholesterol).

- Cholesterol is found only in animal products such as meat and dairy products. Therefore, be sure to select the lean and low-fat versions.
- Plant foods like fruits, vegetables, whole grains, nuts, and legumes (beans) contain no cholesterol. What does that say about what we should be eating more of?
- Exercise elevates the good (HDL) cholesterol in the body.

. . . .

BRAWNIER BONES

Osteoporosis (bone-thinning) commonly affects older adults.

- Encourage strong bones with calcium-rich foods (yogurt, broccoli, beans, almonds, and dark leafy green vegetables).
- Ask your doctor about taking a calcium supplement.
- Get moderate exposure to sunlight (for vitamin D). Don't forget the sunscreen!
- Maintain bone density with regular exercise.
- Limit alcohol, caffeine, sugar, smoking, and phosphorus rich foods (like red meat) which can pull calcium from the system.

. . . .

WONDERFUL WATER

Eight (8-oz) glasses of water daily are recommended for adults.

- It is essential for digestion, eliminating toxins, maintaining normal body temperature, and avoiding constipation.
- Sip slowly and spread your fluids out throughout the day.

- Water may also benefit weight loss. By filling up on more water between meals you can actually reduce hunger.

• • • •

MAGNIFICENT MULTIVITAMINS
Handy for low-cost health insurance, multiple vitamin-mineral supplements can help prevent deficiencies of precious nutrients.

- How to make a selection? Simply choose a 'complete' formula that includes all the common vitamins like A, B-complex, C, D, and E. It should also include the various minerals such as calcium, magnesium, iron, selenium, chromium, molybdenum, manganese, zinc, and possibly others.
- Generic brands are usually fine. Ask your doctor to approve your choices, especially if ill or pregnant.
- Store vitamin supplements safely away from excess heat, cold, sunlight.

• • • •

KIDS & KITCHENS
Encourage children to assist parents when cooking.

- The benefits include quality time together, teaching good eating habits, and learning teamwork and discipline.
- Emphasize safety when working around sharp objects, hot stoves, and electric gadgets.

• • • •

FINICKY EATERS
Got fussy eaters that won't eat their veggies? Try this approach:

- Chop vegetables (such as broccoli and carrots) into small pieces, then conceal them in various dishes.
- Insert veggies into common foods such as pasta sauce, mashed potatoes, rice, sandwiches, burritos, pizza, eggs, soups, casseroles, etc.

FEISTY FOOD CRAVINGS

They may be a signal that you're in need of a certain nutrient that a particular food is noted for.

- For instance, craving a dairy product (like milk or cheese) might signal a need for calcium.
- For more examples, see the nutrient chapter later on in this book for info on foods and their noted nutrients.

• • • •

EFFICIENT EATING

- Good digestion is vital to health and absorption of nutrients.

- Chew foods thoroughly.

- Eat when relaxed and don't rush. If necessary, take a moment to calm yourself first before digging in.

- Never eat until stuffed. Small meals digest much easier. It's better to eat five or six smaller meals in a day rather than three large ones.

- Sip fluids slowly and don't gulp.

• • • •

FRUSTRATING FOOD ALLERGIES

The most common allergens are milk, eggs, nuts, seafood, soy and wheat.

- Symptoms can range from discomforts in the mouth, throat, or stomach to nausea and even loss of consciousness.
- If you suspect a food allergy consult your physician.

• • • •

VEGETARIAN VIRTUES

A healthy lifestyle growing in popularity with millions of followers worldwide.

- People undertake a meatless lifestyle for various reasons, most notably health, religion, or animal rights.
- There are two common types: "Lacto-ovo" vegetarians eat no meat whatsoever, but do include dairy items in their diet. "Vegans" live on plant foods exclusively (fruits, vegetables, grains, legumes, nuts and seeds).
- Most vegetarians tend to be healthier overall compared to the general population. Due to their lifestyle they are known for having fewer problems with cholesterol, blood pressure, and even certain types of cancer. They may live longer as well.

• • • •

WHY WORRY?

Everyone encounters stress, but stress that's out of control can become deadly. Managing stress is the key.

- Be aware that the majority of things which most people worry about never occur.
- Stop worrying about things that are out of your control like the economy, war, and natural disasters. Avoid watching television news reports if they easily upset you.
- Discover healthy forms of relaxation. Like taking walks, reading, listening to music, exercise, positive thinking, religion, or whatever works for you. Remember too, that laughter is great medicine.
- Do you have a quiet place that you can go to in order to relax?

• • • •

NOTE: CONSULT YOUR PHYSICIAN FOR ALL QUESTIONS OR CONCERNS REGARDING THIS TOPIC OR ANY OTHER MATERIAL IN THIS BOOK.

• • • •

NOTABLE NUTRIENTS

Nutrients keep us healthy and prevent ills.

• • • •

The absence of a single nutrient could rob us of our health. They must be acquired thru the foods we eat, which makes food selection very important. Supplements alone seldom do the trick, so efforts to improve eating habits is always the smartest route. Why? Foods contain hidden properties which help the body utilize nutrients more efficiently. That is something which supplements sometimes lack.

• • • •

PROTEIN

- Composes about 20% of entire human body weight. Major building blocks for muscles and organs.
- Sources include all meats, fish, poultry, dairy products, eggs, nuts, legumes (beans), soy, tofu, and seeds (like sunflower).

• • • •

AMINO ACID

- They play central roles both as building blocks of proteins and as intermediates in metabolism. The twenty amino acids that are found within proteins convey a vast array of chemical versatility.
- Humans can produce 10 of the 20 amino acids. The others must be supplied in the food. Failure to obtain enough of even one of the ten essential amino acids, those that we cannot make, results in degradation of the body's proteins (muscles and so forth) to obtain the single amino acid that is needed. Unlike fat and starch, the human body does not store excess amino acids for later use. Therefore, the amino acids must be present in the foods every day.

· · · ·

FAT

- Composes about 15% of entire body weight. A source of energy calories for the body, and helps insulate human organs.
- Fish oils, liquid vegetable oils (like olive oil and canola), flax, avocado, olives, and seeds (such as flax and sunflower) are the recommended sources.

· · · ·

CARBOHYDRATES

- Composes about 2% of our body weight. A chief source of energy and provider of immediate available calories.
- Complex carbs like whole grains, fruit, vegetables, brown rice, nuts, and yams are the recommended sources over simple sugars.

· · · ·

WATER

- Composes about 55% of entire body weight. Regulates body temperature, aids digestion, and flushes out wastes and toxins.
- Bottled water, filtered water, and spring mineral water are the purest selections, and recommended over tap.

· · · ·

FIBER

- Helps to prevent constipation, stabilizing blood sugar levels, and assist in cleaning out the digestive tract.
- Sources of fiber include plant foods such as whole grains, vegetables, fruit, bran, flax, and legumes (beans).

· · · ·

ENZYMES

- Aids digestion and activates various digestive enzymes.
- Found in raw plant foods such as alfalfa sprouts, whole fruit, and vegetables.

. . . .

ANTIOXIDANTS

- Antioxidants are chemicals that can help prevent or slow cell damage and counteract free radicals (a.k.a. cancer-causing properties). There are many antioxidant compounds out there, but the most common dietary ones are vitamins A, C, and E, beta-carotene, selenium and lycopene.
- Natural antioxidants are mainly found in fruits and vegetables, marine plants, and some types of sea creatures that eat marine plants.

. . . .

PHYTONUTRIENTS

- These are compounds found in plants. Not only do phytonutrients offer benefit to the plants but they also provide benefits to those who consume plant food. That's because they have beneficial health promoting properties including antioxidant, anti-inflammatory, and liver health benefits.
- Fruits and vegetables are highly concentrated sources of phytonutrients. Other plant foods such as whole grains, legumes (beans), nuts and seeds, herbs and spices also contain phytonutrients.

. . . .

ELECTROLYTES

- They help regulate our nerve and muscle function, our body's hydration, blood pH, blood pressure, and the rebuilding of damaged tissue. Various mechanisms exist in our body that keep the concentrations of different electrolytes under strict control.

- Common electrolytes include calcium, magnesium, sodium, and potassium. To maintain electrolyte concentrations of our body fluids constant, these must be replaced regularly. Fresh fruits and various vegetables are especially rich in electrolytes.

• • • •

VALUABLE VITAMINS

Vitamins are divided into two groups. The "water soluble" include the B complex, C and bioflavonoids, and the "fat soluble" or vitamins A, D, E, F and K. Water soluble vitamins are measured in milligrams (mgs), and are not stored well by the body. Fat soluble vitamins are measured in international units (IU), and are more readily stored.

Vitamins help convert protein, fats and carbohydrates into energy and aid our metabolism. They assist in tissue formation and repair. Common vitamin deficiencies include Scurvy (vitamin C), Pellagra (niacin), Beriberi (B-1), Rickets (vitamin D), Pernicious anemia (B-12) and night blindness (vitamin A).

Vitamins have no caloric or energy value, but are important to the body as constituents of enzymes, which function as catalysts in nearly all metabolic reactions. Vitamins are not components of body structures, but aid in the building of these features. With few exceptions, the human body cannot manufacture its own vitamins, but is dependent upon foods we eat for supply (an exception is sunshine and vitamin D).

Vitamins make up less than 1% of the human body. They are important as constituents of enzymes and catalysts in metabolic reactions. Best food sources of vitamins in general are milk, fish, vegetables, fruits, whole grains, nuts, seeds and legumes.

• • • •

VITAMIN A

- Important to health of eyes and skin, and also growth and repair of body tissues.

- Sources include vegetables; for example, carrots, broccoli and spinach, plus milk, egg yolks and fish oils.

. . . .

B-VITAMIN COMPLEX

- Important for a healthy nervous system, digestion, appetite, hair and skin; aids protein, fat and carbohydrate metabolism.
- Sources include whole grains such brown rice, whole wheat and wheat germ. Also nuts and brewer's yeast.

. . . .

THIAMINE (B-1)

- Aids protein metabolism, brain function, and carbohydrate digestion. Benefits circulation and red blood cells.
- Sources include brewer's yeast, wheat bran, wheat germ, milk, oats and nuts.

. . . .

RIBOFLAVIN (B-2)

- Important for formation of anti-bodies, cell respiration and metabolism. Also, healthy eyes, skin, nails and hair.
- Sources include milk, whole grains, almonds, and leafy vegetables.

. . . .

NIACIN (B-3)

- Important for proper digestion, circulation and healthy nervous system. Also, protein and carbohydrate metabolism.
- Sources include brown rice, wheat germ, brewer's yeast, nuts, and leafy vegetables.

. . . .

PYRIDOXINE (B-6)

- Important for metabolism of essential fatty acids and protein. Establishes water balance. Benefits energy release of glycogen.
- Sources include bananas, rice, cabbage, milk, nuts and eggs.

• • • •

COBALAMIN (B-12)

- Important for production of red blood cells and prevention of anemia. Benefits brain function and growth. Aids metabolic enzyme processes.
- Sources include meats, dairy products, eggs, yogurt, sauerkraut, soy beans and wheat germ.

• • • •

OROTIC ACID (B-13)

- Important for synthesis of nucleic acid, vital to regeneration process of cells. Suggested as a natural remedy for multiple sclerosis.
- Sources include milk, yogurt, cheese, eggs and soybeans.

• • • •

PANGAMIC ACID (B-15)

- Important for oxygenation of the body, helps regulate fat metabolism, may benefit elevated cholesterol levels, and may help to serves as a detoxifier.
- Sources include brown rice, whole grains, nuts and sunflower seeds.

• • • •

LAETRILE (B-17)

- Suggested in prevention of certain types of cancer. May strengthen the immune system against various malignancies.

- Sources include apple seeds, kernels of fruit like apricots, and millet cereal.

. . . .

BIOTIN

- Important for metabolism of fats and proteins. Benefits healthy hair and growth. Also aids utilization of B complex.
- Sources include brown rice, brewer's yeast, soybeans and whole grains.

. . . .

FOLIC ACID

- Co-worker with other B vitamins in formation of red blood cells. Aids general healing, plus healthy skin and hair.
- Sources include beans, nuts, leafy vegetables, wheat germ and brown rice.

. . . .

CHOLINE

- A component of lecithin which aids fat metabolism and cholesterol control. Stimulates brain function and memory.
- Sources include egg yolks, soybeans, whole kernel corn, brewer's yeast, tofu and legumes.

. . . .

INOSITOL

- Important for metabolism of fats, helps to reduce cholesterol, and is essential to hair growth. Prevents eye dysfunctions.
- Sources include whole grains, rice, brewer's yeast, wheat germ, nuts and milk.

· · · ·

PABA (A.K.A. para-amino-benzoic acid)

- Promotes hair growth and healthy. Aids in prevention of fatigue, eczema and sunburn.
- Sources include milk, eggs, yogurt, whole grains, brewer's yeast and brown rice.

· · · ·

PANTOTHENIC ACID

- Stimulates the adrenal glands. Promotes healing, and benefits the nervous system.
- Sources include whole grains, wheat germ, brown rice, nuts, and eggs.

· · · ·

VITAMIN C

- Strengthens blood vessels, aids resistance to certain infections and virus. Benefits healing of wounds and may help in the prevention of colds and flu.
- Sources include various fruit, citrus fruit, bell peppers, tomatoes, potatoes, papaya and certain vegetables.

· · · ·

VITAMIN D

- Utilization of calcium and phosphorus for bone formation. Plays a role in normal heart action and nervous system.
- Sources include exposure to sunlight, fortified milk, fish oils, and fortified calcium supplements.

· · · ·

VITAMIN E

- Aids normal heart action. Benefits blood clotting, serves as an anti-oxidant, plus cellular respiration and inhibition of aging.
- Sources include wheat germ, egg yolks, whole grains and liquid vegetable oils.

• • • •

VITAMIN F (A.K.A. unsaturated fatty acid)

- Important for lubrication of body organs and blood coagulation. Plays a role in skin and gland maintenance.
- Sources include vegetable oils, soybeans, sunflower seeds, nuts, olives, avocado and egg yolks.

• • • •

VITAMIN K

- Important for formation of prothrombin, a chemical required in blood clotting. Aids normal liver function.
- Sources include egg yolks, green leafy vegetables, yogurt, tomatoes, soy beans and sprouts.

• • • •

VITAMIN P (A.K.A. bioflavonoids)

- An anti-coagulant, benefits the absorption of vitamin C, and helps strengthen capillaries.
- Sources include citrus fruits like oranges, grapefruit, and lemons.

• • • •

VITAMIN T

- Aids in the prevention and correction of certain types of anemia.
- Also known as the "sesame seed factor" since they are top food source.

....

VITAMIN U

● Also called the "cabbage factor" as this is the top food source. Includes sauerkraut and Cole slaw. Aids insulin production, prevention of ulcers; promotes healthy hair, skin and nails.

....

MAGNIFICENT MINERALS

Minerals are divided into two groups. "Macro" which includes calcium, magnesium, phosphorus, potassium, sulfur, chlorine and sodium; and "trace" elements which includes iron, zinc, manganese, iodine, copper, molybdenum, chromium and selenium.

"Macro" minerals are present in larger amounts in the human body than "trace" elements, though both are equally important in health maintenance. Deficiencies of either group can lead to stunted growth, frail conditions, or become linked to various cancers.

Minerals act as catalysts for vitamins, enzymes and amino acids while exerting great influence over mental, physical and emotional states of health. They are especially important to maintenance of bones, cell repair and muscle function.

Vitamins were discovered before minerals, thus made headlines in advance. They, quite simply, stole the health spotlight. A number of people take vitamin supplements, but mistakenly neglect the minerals. Only recently have minerals enjoyed their long overdue popularity, when calcium deficiencies were linked to osteoporosis (bone thinning).

Minerals make up about 5% of entire body weight. They are extremely important for maintenance of bones, muscles, brain and nervous system. Best food sources of minerals generally include dairy, fish, vegetables, fruits, whole grains, nuts, seeds and legumes.

....

CALCIUM

- Maintains strong bones and healthy teeth. Prevents osteoporosis (bone thinning).
- Sources include milk, yogurt, cheese, beans, soy beans, broccoli, dark leafy greens and almonds.

. . . .

PHOSPHORUS

- Works in conjunction with calcium in bone and teeth formation.
- Sources include meats, dairy, eggs, beans, nuts, whole grains, and brewer's yeast.

. . . .

MAGNESIUM

- Important for proper functioning of nervous system, enzyme activator and utilization of major nutrients.
- Sources include whole grains, nuts, leafy vegetables, soybeans and dolomite supplements.

. . . .

POTASSIUM

- Important for proper function of muscles, nerves, heart and kidneys. Helps maintain water balance.
- Sources include most fruits (especially bananas), various vegetables, potatoes and tomatoes.

. . . .

SODIUM

- Works with potassium in fluid balance, health of nervous system, and plays a role in muscle control.
- Sources include table salt, sea salt, celery, seafood, ocean kelp

(seaweed), soy sauce and processed foods.

· · · ·

IRON

- Important for prevention of anemia. Aids hemoglobin formation and oxygen transport from blood to the tissues.
- Sources include oats, spinach, raisins, beef liver and blackstrap molasses.

· · · ·

SULPHUR

- Important for maintenance of hair, skin and nails. Aids insulin production, metabolism, and collagen synthesis.
- Sources include cabbage, Cole slaw, eggs, sauerkraut, Brussels sprouts, onions and garlic.

· · · ·

CHLORINE

- Aids production of hydrochloric acid (HCL) for healthy digestion.
- Sources include seafood, sea salt, kelp, rye flour, and olives.

· · · ·

MANGANESE

- Important for skeletal development, muscle coordination, enzyme activator and carbohydrate metabolism.
- Sources include whole wheat, wheat bran, nuts, beans, pineapple, black pepper and egg yolks.

· · · ·

ZINC

- Component of insulin. Aids healing, metabolism and activates enzymes.
- Sources include corn, mushrooms, nuts, sunflower seeds, whole grains, brewer's yeast, and oysters.

• • • •

COPPER

- Important for formation of red blood cells, bone formation and production of RNA.
- Sources include whole grains, nuts, beans, raisins, blackstrap molasses and seafood.

• • • •

CHROMIUM

- Important for insulin effectiveness and glucose tolerance factor. Aids energy metabolism, and enzyme activity.
- Sources include whole wheat, nuts, brewer's yeast, nutritional yeast, wheat germ and seafood.

• • • •

IODINE

- Important for thyroid function, energy, growth, mentality, speech, and fat metabolism. Also, healthy hair, nails, skin.
- Sources include ocean kelp (seaweed), iodized salt, sea salt, ocean fish and seafood.

• • • •

MOLYBDENUM

- Utilization of iron, oxidation of fats, enzyme activator and component. Sources include whole grains, nuts, beans, and green leafy vegetables.

. . . .

SELENIUM

- An anti-oxidant. Aids tissue elasticity. Works with vitamin E for normal body growth and fertility.
- Sources include whole grains, seaweed and various seafood.

. . . .

LITHIUM

- Commonly used in treatment of manic-depression. Sold as pharmaceutical prescription.
- Natural sources include most seafood and ocean kelp.

. . . .

COBALT

- Maintains red blood cells and prevents anemia. Component of vitamin B-12 (cobalamin).
- Sources include meats, milk, eggs, yogurt, seafood and green leafy vegetables.

. . . .

VANADIUM

- Plays a role in inhibiting cholesterol formation. Benefits bone, tooth and cartilage development.
- Sources include seafood, whole grains, vegetable oils and ocean kelp.

. . . .

SILICON

- Plays a role in health of connective tissues and health of tendons, cartilage and blood vessels.
- Sources include hard drinking water, buckwheat flour, oats and various plant fibers.

. . . .

NICKEL

- May play a role in RNA and DNA, plus hormone and glucose metabolism.
- Sources include whole grains, beans, seeds, various vegetables and seafood.

. . . .

FLUORINE

- Works with calcium in formation of bones & teeth. Considered toxic in high (synthetic) amounts.
- Sources include seafood, cheese, tea, toothpaste and fluoridated drinking water.

. . . .

GERMANIUM

- Plays a role in strengthening the immune system for resistance to various forms of illness.
- Sources include garlic, onions, ginseng, ocean kelp and various seafood.

. . . .

STRONTIUM

- May be involved in proper bone growth and prevention of tooth decay.

- Found primarily in various ocean sources like kelp (seaweed) and seafood.

. . . .

TIN

- Plays a role in hemoglobin synthesis and growth rate. Excesses from industry sources can be toxic.
- Sources include stannous fluoride toothpastes, kelp and seafood.

. . . .

NOTE: CONSULT YOUR PHYSICIAN FOR ALL QUESTIONS OR CONCERNS REGARDING THIS TOPIC OR ANY OTHER MATERIAL IN THIS BOOK.

. . . .

NOTE: NOT INTENDED TO PRESCRIBE OR DIAGNOSE. CONSULT YOUR PHYSICIAN FOR ALL HEALTH CONCERNS INCLUDING MEDICAL TREATMENTS, MEDICATIONS, DIETARY ALTERATIONS, VITAMIN SUPPLEMENTS, AND BEFORE STARTING A FITNESS PROGRAM.

MOMENTOUS MEAL STARTERS

Breakfast, lunch and dinner.

• • • •

BREAKFAST BUDDIES
Forget the sugary doughnuts and high-fat bacon or sausage!

- Traditional breakfasts are typically high in fat and sugar, and often lacking in fiber or other nutrients.
- Start your morning right with a healthy protein food like a poached or hard-boiled egg, or low-fat yogurt.
- Include some whole fruit or 100% juice if desired.
- Add a whole grain item such as whole wheat toast, bran muffin, multi-grain bagel, or high-fiber cereal like oatmeal or bran flakes.

• • • •

Recommended:

- Poached or hard-boiled egg
- Veggie-stuffed omelet with low-fat cheese.
- Cholesterol-free egg whites or Egg Beaters.
- Whole grain toast, bagel, or English muffin.
- High-fiber cereal like bran flakes or oatmeal
- Whole grain waffles topped with fruit
- Bran muffin or granola cereal bar
- Low-fat yogurt or non-dairy soy yogurt
- Whole fruit such as grapefruit, berries, or prunes
- Tomato juice or V-8 juice
- 100% fruit juice (no added sugar)
- Green tea or herbal tea
- Decaf coffee served black.
- Low-fat milk or non-dairy milk made from soy, rice, or almond.
- 100% Fruit preserves (no added sugar)

Not Recommended:

- Fried or scrambled eggs
- Ham and cheese omelet
- Bacon, ham, or sausage
- Fried potatoes
- Biscuits and gravy
- Buttermilk pancakes w/butter and syrup
- French toast w/butter and syrup
- White bread toast
- Sugary cereal
- Doughnuts, pastry, or Danish.
- Whole milk
- Juices with added sugar
- Coffee with cream and sugar
- Butter
- Jelly (preserves with added sugar)

• • • •

LAVISH LUNCH

Beware of common fast- food lunches (like burger & fries, pizza and fried chicken) which are typically high in fat & calories.

- Lite and healthy considerations include tossed salads, vegetable soup, bean burrito, or a sandwich of lean turkey, tuna, or low-fat cheese on whole grain bread.
- Low-fat cottage cheese is a versatile lunch cornerstone. It can be topped with various fruit or vegetables. Also consider yogurt.

• • • •

DELIGHTFUL DINNERS

Emphasize lean entrees such as fish fillets or skinless poultry.

- Or try some vegetarian dishes featuring cholesterol-free beans and rice or various soy foods.

- Lite and healthy side dishes include corn, beans, brown rice, peas, lentils, sweet potato, polenta, couscous, and whole grain bread.
- Nourishment is incomplete without veggies (broccoli, spinach, collards, kale, asparagus, carrots, cauliflower, cabbage, etc.). Try as side dish or tossed salad.

• • • •

NOTE: CONSULT YOUR PHYSICIAN FOR ALL QUESTIONS OR CONCERNS REGARDING THIS TOPIC OR ANY OTHER MATERIAL IN THIS BOOK.

• • • •

NOTE: NOT INTENDED TO PRESCRIBE OR DIAGNOSE. CONSULT YOUR PHYSICIAN FOR ALL HEALTH CONCERNS INCLUDING MEDICAL TREATMENTS, MEDICATIONS, DIETARY ALTERATIONS, VITAMIN SUPPLEMENTS, AND BEFORE STARTING A FITNESS PROGRAM.

CHOLESTEROL CONTENT OF FOODS

Cholesterol levels "above 200" are a warning sign that dietary improvements are in order.

• • • •

Notice on the list below that animal products (meat and dairy) contain cholesterol while plant foods have none. So, in order to naturally control our cholesterol what does that tell us about which foods we should be eating more of, and less of?

- Cheeseburger (Regular) +45
- Pepperoni Pizza (Two Slice) +60
- Bacon (Two Slice) +70
- Fried Chicken (Breast) +111
- Whole Milk +34
- Cheese (Slice) +18
- Butter (Tsp) +31
- Chocolate Éclair +152
- Grains +0
- Legumes +0
- Fruits +0
- Vegetables +0
- Beans +0
- Tofu +0
- Nuts +0
- Seeds +0
- Sprouts +0
- Herbs +0

DO-IT-RIGHT DIET ARRANGER

This simple list can become a useful tool in the pursuit of eating right, preventing ills, maintaining normal weight, and living longer.

• • • •

- It will help to ensure that the user will have an adequate intake of protective nutrients like vitamins, minerals, fiber, anti-oxidants, Phyto-nutrients, and natural enzymes.
- Additionally, it will help individuals to keep the less healthy foods (those loaded with fat, saturated fat, sugar and salt) at a minimum.

USE FREQUENTLY

- Vegetables
- Whole Fruits
- Whole Grains
- Legumes (Beans)
- Soy Foods
- Tofu
- Bran And Psyllium Fiber
- Nuts (Dry-Roasted)
- Sunflower Seeds
- Sprouts
- Flax
- Sea Vegetables (Seaweed)
- Herbs
- Green Tea

• • • •

USE MODERATELY

- Fish Fillet
- Skinless Poultry

- Low-Fat Dairy Items
- Egg Yolks
- Potatoes
- Olive Oil
- Processed Grains
- Multi-Grain Items
- Pretzels
- Crackers
- Popcorn
- Vinegar
- Sea Salt
- Black Tea

• • • •

USE SPARINGLY OR AVOID

- Red Meats (Beef And Pork)
- Whole Dairy Products
- Shellfish
- Butter
- Margarine
- Lard
- Trans Fats (Hydrogenated Oils)
- Snack Chips
- Sugar
- All Sweeteners
- White Flour
- Table Salt
- Food Additives
- Coffee

• • • •

NOTE: CONSULT YOUR PHYSICIAN FOR ALL QUESTIONS OR CONCERNS REGARDING THIS TOPIC OR ANY OTHER MATERIAL IN THIS BOOK.

• • • •

NOTE: NOT INTENDED TO PRESCRIBE OR DIAGNOSE. CONSULT YOUR PHYSICIAN FOR ALL HEALTH CONCERNS INCLUDING MEDICAL TREATMENTS, MEDICATIONS, DIETARY ALTERATIONS, VITAMIN SUPPLEMENTS, AND BEFORE STARTING A FITNESS PROGRAM.

CALORIE COMBUSTORS

Regular exercise is an important key to health for lowering cholesterol, improving circulation, relieving depression, improving heart health, and increasing life spans. The chart below shows how many calories various physical activities will burn off in one thirty-minute session.

• • • •

ACTIVITY -—CALORIES BURNED

- Aerobic (low impact) -192
- Ballroom dancing -96
- Cleaning -114
- Hiking -214
- In-line skating -192
- Line dancing -312
- Running (9-minute mile) -360
- Sex -85
- Skiing (cross-country) -222
- Skiing (downhill) -183
- Stair-stepping -206
- Swimming (slow crawl) -237
- Tennis -204
- Walking (20-minute mile) -150
- Yoga -100

• • • •

NOTE: CONSULT YOUR PHYSICIAN FOR ALL QUESTIONS OR CONCERNS REGARDING THIS TOPIC OR ANY OTHER MATERIAL IN THIS BOOK.

• • • •

POTENT PROTEINS

The building block of life.

• • • •

- Protein is composed of amino acids and is essential for muscle growth and tissue repair.
- Complete protein is especially abundant in all animal foods (meats and dairy products).
- Protein-rich sources from the plant kingdom include: legumes (beans), nuts, whole grains, soy foods, tofu, and seeds (like sunflower).

• • • •

RED MEAT MAKEOVER
Tips to help cut back on cholesterol.

- For less saturated fat select lean cuts of beef, pork and lamb.
- Trim and discard all visible fat.
- Beware of high-fat gravies.
- Broiling, grilling, and roasting are low-fat methods recommended for preparing meat.

• • • •

POPULAR POULTRY
Versatile and a low-fat protein;

• Reduce the saturated fat content by removing and discarding the skins. The skins are also unhealthy because they store toxins.

• Turkey has more protein than chicken, and less fat than beef and pork.

• White meat has less fat than dark.

- Broiling, grilling, and roasting are low-fat methods for preparing poultry.

· · · ·

FABULOUS FISH

A low-fat food, choose fish fillets more often.

- Fish contain Omega-3 fatty acids which may lower risk of heart disease. It is found in fish such as lake trout, salmon, mackerel, herring, sardines, and albacore tuna.
- Grilling, baking, and poaching are low-fat methods for preparing fish.

· · · ·

MAJESTIC MILK

A beverage that is rich in protein and calcium.

- Calcium is valuable for healthy bones and teeth. Adults may not need milk since their bones have stopped growing, but children do.
- Select low-fat milk over whole milk. Or, try cholesterol-free non-dairy milk made from soy, almond or rice.
- Some people are allergic to milk (a.k.a. lactose intolerance). Symptoms can include headaches, nausea, indigestion, diarrhea, stomach cramps, or gas.

· · · ·

CLASSY CHEESE

Such a versatile food for meals and snacks.

- Like most dairy products, cheese is a good source of protein and calcium.
- Read labels and select low-fat or reduced-fat options. Whole cheese is high in saturated fat which can raise cholesterol.
- For cholesterol-free alternatives, try non-dairy cheese imitations

made from soy, tofu, rice, or almond.

• • • •

YIPPEE FOR YOGURT

This food has soared in popularity. Here's why:

- An excellent source of protein and calcium, and considered easier to digest than milk.
- Select versions that contain probiotics or "active yogurt cultures". This is a healthy bacterium that actually aids digestion and boosts our immune system.
- Choose low-fat or fat-free versions. Beware of commercial varieties with a high sugar content.

• • • •

EXCELLENT EGGS

An excellent source of high-quality complete protein.

- When frying cook eggs in pure liquid vegetable oil (like olive oil or canola) or a low-cholesterol margarine rather than butter.
- Poached and hard-boiled eggs have less fat than fried and scrambled.
- Serve eggs with healthy extras such as "whole grain" versions of toast, muffin, cereal, or else yogurt or fruit. Do so instead of serving with high-fat bacon, sausage or pancakes.

• • • •

OMELETS

That grand gourmet food of breakfasts...

- For a healthier version stuff an omelet with more low-fat vegetables and less high-fat meat and cheese.
- Select from wholesome veggies such as mushroom, bell pepper, onion, tomato, broccoli, spinach, garlic, asparagus, etc.
- Fry omelets in pure vegetable oil (like olive oil or canola oil) or else a low-cholesterol margarine rather than butter.

41

- Serve omelets with healthy extras like whole grain toast and fruit.

. . . .

LUSCIOUS LEGUMES
These are foods that grow in a pod and include beans, peas, lentils, and peanuts

- Legumes contain the most protein of any plant food, and are popular as meat alternatives around the globe. They are also a favorite among vegetarians.
- In addition to protein they are low-fat, cholesterol-free, and a decent source of fiber and calcium.

. . . .

BEANS
Part of the legume family.

- They are low-fat and a good source of protein and fiber. Serve as a cholesterol-free meat substitute if so desired.
- Use as a side dish or add to soups, burritos, salads, chili, eggs, casseroles, stir-fries, etc.
- Cut the fat content in canned versions by ignoring those made with pork, bacon, or lard.

. . . .

SOY FOODS
These are foods that are made from soybeans.

- Sold commercially, they are popular imitators of common foods like meats (burger patties, sausage, meatballs, deli slices, and hot dogs) and also dairy items (cheese, milk and ice cream).

- Commonly used as meat alternatives, most soy foods are cholesterol-free and protein-rich. Read nutrition labels for fat and sugar content of certain commercially prepared products.

- Frequent use of soy foods used in place of meat may benefit cholesterol levels and help reduce certain cancer risks.

••••

TOFU
Made from soy beans, tofu is protein-rich and low-fat.

- Try as a meat substitute in stir-frying, soups, burritos, casseroles, omelets, and more.
- Tofu is also used to make cholesterol-free desserts.
- A bland food on its own, however, tofu absorbs flavors amazingly well. Enhance its flavor and improve the taste considerably with herbs, spices, sauces and dressings.

••••

NUTRITIOUS NUTS
A powerhouse of nourishment.

- Nuts offer protein, fiber, B-vitamins, and various trace minerals including magnesium, manganese, copper and zinc.
- Try as a snack between meals to help stabilize energy levels, especially for those late afternoon blues.
- Nuts and nut butters are high in fat calories, so be sure to use in moderation.

••••

SENSATIONAL SEEDS
Like nuts, seeds are also a powerhouse of nourishment.

- Seeds are a good source of protein, various vitamins, and minerals.
- Try a handful of sunflower seeds or pumpkin seeds as a snack between meals to help stabilize energy levels. Use sparingly or else they can become fattening.
- Flax seeds contain alpha-linolenic acid, the healthy omega-3 fatty

acid notably found in fish oil which may benefit heart health.

- Seeds contain oils, so they should be stored in a refrigerator or cool dark place to prevent rancidity.

. . . .

CHA CHA CHILI

Create your own "low-fat, high-fiber" chili recipe.

- The key creating chili with a lower saturated fat content is to use less meat and more beans. This step will also grant you a lot more fiber.
- Chili can be made with a combination of several beans such as kidney, pinto, black, red, white, garbanzo, or others.
- Serve chili with "whole grain" versions of bread or crackers.

. . . .

CLASSY CASSEROLES

The key to healthier casseroles.

- Reduce the total fat calories by using less meat and cheese, then substitute vegetables and/or beans instead.
- Great additions to casseroles include veggies such broccoli, spinach, asparagus, mushroom, cauliflower, kale, collards, cabbage and bell pepper.
- You can use beans of all types (red, green, black, or white), peas, lentils, tofu, and whole grains like oats or brown rice.
- Cut the fat but not the flavor by adding tomato sauce or salsa, then season with various spices but go light on the salt.

. . . .

NOTE: CONSULT YOUR PHYSICIAN FOR ALL QUESTIONS OR CONCERNS REGARDING THIS TOPIC OR ANY OTHER MATERIAL IN THIS BOOK.

. . . .

WHOLESOME WHOLE GRAINS

Hurray for the mighty grains!

. . . .

- Whole grains include unrefined versions wheat, rye, oats, barley, brown rice, millet, buckwheat, and whole kernel corn among others which may be lesser known in the U.S. but not in other parts of the world.
- Most whole grains are a prominent source of fiber, B-vitamins, trace minerals, complex carbohydrates and some protein.
- Look for whole grain versions of bread, cereal, muffins, bagels, noodles, rice, tortillas, pancakes, waffles and flour at your grocers.
- Because not all grains are "whole" be sure to read the nutrition label to ensure you are actually getting a whole grain.

. . . .

BENEVOLENT BREAD

For toast or sandwiches

- Whole grain bread offers more fiber, B-vitamins, vitamin E, and trace elements than refined white flour bread.
- 100% whole wheat is generally the preferred choice.
- Don't be deceived! A bread marked as "wheat bread" or "multi-grain" does not necessarily mean whole grain. Read the nutrition label to ensure you are getting a true whole grain product. Some loaves are made up mostly of white flour and only contain a small portion of whole grain flour.

Generally, the heavier and darker the bread the greater the nutrient value. Whole grain breads will also contain more fiber than white bread.

. . . .

CRUNCHY CEREAL

For kids and adults alike.

- When buying cereal seek those that contain the most fiber and the least amount of sugar. Compare labels to similar items for the smartest choice.
- Choose a whole grain or high-fiber version such as bran flakes, whole wheat, or hot oatmeal.
- Serve cereal with low-fat milk or non-dairy milk made from soy, almond or rice. They are cholesterol-free.
- Top cereal with real fruit instead of sugar. Select from options such as sliced bananas, berries, peaches, or raisins.

• • • •

TOAST
That all-time breakfast favorite.

- Choose "whole grain" versions of bread, bagels, or English muffin.
- Select a reduced-fat spread. Or, try low-fat cream cheese.
- For jams and jellies, select all-natural preserves, made with 100% real fruit (no added sugars).

• • • •

RICE
As a side dish instead of potatoes or else a complete meal.

- Brown rice is a good source of fiber and is recommended over common polished white rice.
- For a complete meal, top a bed of cooked rice with healthy options such as veggies, beans, peas, lentils, nuts, or tofu.
- Create a healthy dessert by mixing leftover rice with fruit.

• • • •

PASTA
Mama Mia! Who doesn't like pasta?

- Choose whole grain versions of noodles. Read labels to be sure.
- Cut calories and cholesterol by topping your noodles with more vegetables and fewer meatballs.
- Be creative by adding various veggies to pasta sauce. Select from options such as mushroom, bell pepper, zucchini, broccoli, spinach, asparagus, beans, lentils, garlic, and onion.
- Go light when adding cheese, or use a low-fat version.

• • • •

CRISPY CRACKERS
Such a great snack or even a complete meal.

- Choose whole grain crackers such as whole wheat, rye, or multi-grain.
- Serve crackers with a low-fat cheese or cream cheese, humus, bean dip, or all-natural peanut butter.
- Crackers are also great when served with raw veggies such as broccoli, cauliflower, carrot, celery, olive, bell pepper, mushroom, onion, and tomato.

• • • •

PLUMP PANCAKES AND WAFFLES
Traditionally they can be a real belly buster. Here's how to improve quality.

- Select a whole grain or multi-grain version.
- Cut calories by topping with real fruit instead of butter, syrup or whipped cream.
- Add real fruit toppings such as berries, sliced bananas, or raisins.

• • • •

PUFFY POPPED CORN
Popcorn can be a wholesome snack and good source of fiber.

- Beware of high-calorie popcorn flavorings including butter, cheese, caramel and sweetened kettle corn.
- Go light when adding salt. Create flavor by adding herbs and spices.

Try various blends like Italian seasoning or others.

- The oil-free method of air-popped corn is best.

• • • •

BRAN MUFFINS

A healthier alternative to doughnuts at breakfast, and good source of fiber.

- Use bran muffins in moderation, for they do contain fat and sugar.
- Try a bran muffin with green tea, yogurt, an egg or fruit at breakfast.

• • • •

MARVELOUS MACARONI & CHEESE

- Use whole grain noodles instead of common white macaroni.
- Reduce the amount of cheese or select a version lower in fat.
- Instead of whole milk use low-fat milk or a non-dairy version made from soy, almond or rice. They are cholesterol-free.
- Boost nutrition by adding some peas or chopped broccoli.
- Replace the butter with olive oil.

• • • •

NOTE: CONSULT YOUR PHYSICIAN FOR ALL QUESTIONS OR CONCERNS REGARDING THIS TOPIC OR ANY OTHER MATERIAL IN THIS BOOK.

• • • •

NOTE: NOT INTENDED TO PRESCRIBE OR DIAGNOSE. CONSULT YOUR PHYSICIAN FOR ALL HEALTH CONCERNS INCLUDING MEDICAL TREATMENTS, MEDICATIONS, DIETARY ALTERATIONS, VITAMIN SUPPLEMENTS, AND BEFORE STARTING A FITNESS PROGRAM.

VALUABLE VEGGIES

It's difficult to be healthy without them.

• • • •

- Vegetables offer protective nutrients such as vitamins, minerals, anti-oxidants, beta-carotene (a form of vitamin A), and Phyto-nutrients (plant nutrients).
- Researchers will testify that a vegetable-rich diet can potentially help prevent many ravaging ills such as cancers, heart disease, and premature aging.
- For optimum nutrition be sure to select a rainbow of colored vegetables for your diet.

• • • •

VERSATILE VEGGIES
Boost your daily nutrition by adding more vegetables to common foods.

- Vegetables can be added to pasta sauce, mashed potatoes, sandwiches, rice, burritos, pizza, omelets, soups, and casseroles.
- Steaming and grilling are advocated for low-fat cooking. When stir-frying cook veggies in pure olive oil.
- Got fussy eaters that won't eat their veggies? Try this approach! Chop vegetables into small pieces, then conceal them in various dishes.

• • • •

GREAT GREENS
Noted for their highly nutritious and healing properties.

- Dark colored leafy greens include vegetables such as spinach, collards, turnip greens, mustard greens, kale, cabbage, and Romaine lettuce.
- They are low-fat and a rich source of nutrients including vitamin A, calcium, and fiber.
- Leafy greens make a fine side dish, tossed into soups and salads, and

added to sandwiches.

. . . .

CELESTIAL CRUCIFEROUS VEGGIES
Much acclaimed by science as a potential cancer preventive.

- Members of the cabbage family, they are so named as their stalk resembles a cross.
- They include broccoli, cabbage, kale, cauliflower, turnips, collard greens, and Brussels sprouts.

. . . .

OPULENT ORANGE VEGGIES
Medical researchers have discovered the amazing anti-oxidant powers of beta-carotene in orange-colored vegetables.

- Such foods are known to help boost the immune system. They include yams, squash, pumpkin and carrots.
- These vegetables improve our night vision, and may help prevent certain cancers, skin disorders, premature aging, plus a host of degenerative ills.

. . . .

SENSATIONAL SALADS
For optimum health choose salads that contain a variety of vegetables.

- Think beyond ordinary lettuce and tomato salads. Try adding broccoli, cauliflower, spinach, kale, collard greens, cabbage, olives, onion, or other favorites.
- Select low-fat dressings for tossed salads.
- Or, make your own natural salad dressing with olive oil and balsamic vinegar. Add various herbs or spices for flavor if desired.
- Beware of high-fat extras in common salads such as bacon, ham, cheese, egg yolks, mayo, and sour cream.

SUPER SLAW

Cabbage is a cruciferous veggie known to help prevent certain types of cancers.

- Make a Cole slaw mix featuring grated green cabbage, chopped onions, carrots, and some chopped parsley.
- Add a low-fat mayo or apple cider vinegar, and some lemon juice or yellow mustard. Flavor with salt and pepper and maybe a light amount of sugar if needed.

· · · ·

GRAND GARLIC AND ONIONS

Popular with chefs around the globe because they add so much flavor to foods.

- Staples of ancient civilizations, they are world famous as folk remedies.
- Touted as immune system boosters which may help prevent certain types of cancers, stroke, and even colds and flu.

· · · ·

TATER TOPPERS

As alternatives to high-fat butter, sour cream, or cheese.

- Try low-fat toppings on baked potatoes such as salsa, pasta sauce, plain yogurt, mustard, catsup, or herbs.
- Create an entire meal by burying a baked potato in veggies. Consider options such as broccoli, cauliflower, mushrooms, beans, corn, spinach, asparagus, bell peppers, onions, or other favorites.
- Yams and sweet potatoes are nutritionally superior to white potatoes.

· · · ·

MAJESTIC MASHED POTATOES

Here's how to cut the fat content and boost nutrition.

- Cook and mash whole potatoes in regular fashion, but keep the skins intact. The under layer houses many nutrients. Be sure to wash the outer skin before using.
- Instead of mixing potatoes with whole milk use low-fat milk, vegetable broth, or soy milk.
- Instead of butter try topping with herbs and spices.
- Boost nutrition by mixing in some finely chopped broccoli.

• • • •

FRISKY FRENCH FRIES

Beware of those traditional high-fat deep-fried versions.

- Bake sliced potatoes in an oven on a tray coated with light amount of vegetable oil or a spray oil.
- Go easy on salt. Flavor with a variety of herbs and spices.
- Baked till golden brown.

• • • •

PIZZA PIZZAZZ

Cut the fat calories by topping pizza with more vegetables and less meat.

- Pile on the healthy veggies such as mushroom, bell pepper, onion, broccoli, spinach, tomato, olives, asparagus, garlic, or other favorites.
- A whole grain crust is more nutritious than a white flour crust. Check around for availability (grocers may carry them but not delivery chains).
- For less fat beware of 'double cheese' versions.
- For fewer calories choose 'thin crust' over 'deep dish'.

• • • •

SAVORY SOUP

Nourishing soup should overflow with an abundance of hearty vegetables.

- Get creative and select from veggie options such as broccoli, carrot, cauliflower, asparagus, onion, kale, spinach, cabbage, celery, garlic, peas, lentils, corn, beans, or other favorites.

- Serve soup with 'whole grain' versions of bread or crackers.

· · · ·

CREATIVE CASSEROLES

Cut calories in casseroles by substituting a portion of the high-fat meats and cheeses with vegetables.

- Select from healthy options such as broccoli, onion, cauliflower, asparagus, carrot, spinach, cabbage, celery, garlic, peas, lentils, corn, kale, or beans.
- In place of fatty red meats, you could also use other low-fat ingredients for casseroles such as skinless turkey, tuna, or reduced-fat cheese.

· · · ·

NOTE: CONSULT YOUR PHYSICIAN FOR ALL QUESTIONS OR CONCERNS REGARDING THIS TOPIC OR ANY OTHER MATERIAL IN THIS BOOK.

· · · ·

NOTE: NOT INTENDED TO PRESCRIBE OR DIAGNOSE. CONSULT YOUR PHYSICIAN FOR ALL HEALTH CONCERNS INCLUDING MEDICAL TREATMENTS, MEDICATIONS, DIETARY ALTERATIONS, VITAMIN SUPPLEMENTS, AND BEFORE STARTING A FITNESS PROGRAM.

Consuming more fresh fruit instead of high-calorie snacks can benefit waistlines.

• • • •

- Most fruits are low in fat and sodium and are a good source of vitamin C, potassium, fiber, and natural carbohydrates.
- Beware of commercial fruits with added sugars. For example, canned fruits, dried fruits, and juice concentrates.

• • • •

CITRUS AND C

Oranges, grapefruit, lemon, limes and tangerines are sources of vitamin C.

- Vitamin C boosts our immune system and prevents scurvy, infection, certain cancers, and eases stress.
- Some reports suggest the vitamin C found in fruit may help prevent seasonal colds and flu.

• • • •

BANANA BOUNTY

Great on breakfast cereal and as between meal snacks.

- Bananas are a quick energy, natural-carbohydrate food that's low in fat and sodium.
- They are rich in potassium, an electrolyte and mineral valuable for muscle and brain function that also helps eliminate excess sodium in the system which benefits blood pressure.

• • • •

BRAZEN BERRIES

Blueberries, blackberries, strawberries, and cranberries.

- Most berries are rich in antioxidants which may help in the prevention of various cancers.
- Blueberries contain resveratrol, believed to help reduce risk of heart disease, certain cancers, and may benefit eye health and urinary tract.
- Try cranberry juice to help cleanse the kidneys. Avoid those with added sugars.

· · · ·

ANGELIC AVOCADO

Did you know they are classified as a fruit?

- They're rich in unsaturated fatty acids which are good for healthy skin, hair, eyes, and internal organs.
- Try sliced avocado on sandwiches or in salads.
- Mashed ripe avocados make a fine dip for crackers.
- The avocado is NOT fat-free, so use in moderation.

· · · ·

TOMATO TALLY

Yes, tomatoes are actually a fruit.

- The tomato is a low-fat food and a good source of lycopene, which can help prevent some cancers.
- They may also help reduce blood pressure due to their potassium content.
- A fine addition to sandwiches and salads, and who doesn't like tomato sauce on their pasta or pizza?

· · · ·

NOTE: CONSULT YOUR PHYSICIAN FOR ALL QUESTIONS OR CONCERNS REGARDING THIS TOPIC OR ANY OTHER MATERIAL IN THIS BOOK.

· · · ·

NOTE: NOT INTENDED TO PRESCRIBE OR DIAGNOSE. CONSULT YOUR PHYSICIAN FOR ALL HEALTH CONCERNS INCLUDING MEDICAL TREATMENTS, MEDICATIONS, DIETARY ALTERATIONS, VITAMIN SUPPLEMENTS, AND BEFORE STARTING A FITNESS PROGRAM.

SENSIBLE SANDWICHES & SUBS

It's amazing what two slices of bread can provide.

• • • •

- To control the saturated fat content shy away from cold cuts such as ham, bologna and salami. Instead select lean fillers such as tuna fish, skinless chicken and turkey, low-fat cheese, or humus (bean dip).
- Add healthy veggies such as leafy greens, tomato, onion, mushroom, olive, sprouts, and bell pepper.
- Mustard is the preferred condiment. It's low-fat (unlike mayo) and sugar-free (unlike ketchup).
- Serve on whole grain or multi-grain versions of bread instead of white flour bread.

• • • •

BETTER BURGERS
How to nutritionally improve that fast food favorite.

- Select lean patties made from poultry or tuna in place of fatty beef.
- Or try veggie patties made from grains, veggies or soy. You could also grill a large Portobello mushroom instead.
- Boost nutrition by adding veggies such as various leafy greens, tomato, onions, and mushrooms. Or, try adding Cole slaw!
- For a cheeseburger use a low-fat version of cheese.
- For better nutrition serve patties on a whole grain or multi-grain bun.
- Beware of high-fat extras like mayo, bacon, fries and shakes. Instead, serve burgers with beans, corn, or tossed salad.

• • • •

FLAMING FRANKS
Plump up the nutritional quality of your pups.

- Select lean hot dogs made from turkey, chicken, or soy.

- Add low-fat toppings like tomato, onion, sauerkraut, pickles, and mustard.
- For better nutrition choose 'whole grain' versions of buns or sub rolls.
- Beware of high-fat fries and shakes. Serve pups with healthy extras like beans, corn, salad, or Cole slaw.

• • • •

BOUNDLESS BURRITOS & TACOS
Add zest to these souths of the border favorites.

- Use lean fillers such as turkey, tuna, low-fat cheese, brown rice, and lard-free refried beans.
- Add healthy veggies such as leafy greens, tomato, onion, bell pepper, mushrooms, broccoli, or spinach.
- Flavor with salsa instead of high-fat sour cream.
- Boost nutrition by serving on 'whole grain' tortilla shells.

• • • •

POPULAR PEANUT BUTTER
For kids and adults alike.

- Select an all-natural version of nut butter (no added oils or sugar).
- For jam or jelly, choose all-natural preserves made with real fruit and no added sugars.
- Add ripe sliced banana instead of jam if desired.
- Serve on whole grain or multi-grain versions of bread.

• • • •

TEMPTING TOASTED CHEESE
Subtle changes can improve nutritional quality.

- Choose a reduced-fat version of cheese. Or, try the assortment of non-dairy, cholesterol-free imitation cheeses made from soy, tofu, almond or tapioca.
- Boost nutrition with a whole grain or multi-grain version of bread.

- Use a reduced-fat spread instead of butter.
- Add a slice of real tomato instead of high-fat bacon.

• • • •

BLAZING BLT SANDWICH

For a slimmer version.

- Try cholesterol-free soy bacon (sold in health stores). Imitation bacon bits can suffice as well.
- Use low-fat mayo instead of traditional mayonnaise.
- Serve on whole grain or multi-grain bread along with fresh lettuce and tomato.

• • • •

SUPER SLOPPY JOE'S

Creative fun within a bun.

- Save on fat calories and substitute lean ground turkey for ground beef.
- Or, try a cholesterol-free imitation meat substitute made from lentils or soy protein (sold in health retailers).
- Boost nutrition by serving on "whole grain" versions of buns.
- Serve your Joe's with a tossed salad, corn or beans.

• • • •

NOTE: CONSULT YOUR PHYSICIAN FOR ALL QUESTIONS OR CONCERNS REGARDING THIS TOPIC OR ANY OTHER MATERIAL IN THIS BOOK.

• • • •

NOTE: NOT INTENDED TO PRESCRIBE OR DIAGNOSE. CONSULT YOUR PHYSICIAN FOR ALL HEALTH CONCERNS INCLUDING MEDICAL TREATMENTS, MEDICATIONS, DIETARY ALTERATIONS, VITAMIN SUPPLEMENTS, AND BEFORE STARTING A FITNESS PROGRAM.

HEALTH HAZARDS

SWEET SUGAR
The Sour Truth

- White refined sugar offers no nutrition other than carbohydrates and has been linked to obesity, hypoglycemia, diabetes, hyperactivity, and tooth decay.
- The average American eats more than fifty pounds of this stuff each year. That's over a pound per week! Consider the weight you could potentially lose by avoiding it or cutting back.
- Natural sugars (like honey and brown sugar) not much better. Though slightly higher in nutrients, they are high in calories which can burst a waistline and wreak havoc upon blood sugar levels.
- To satisfy a sweet tooth, switch to whole fruit. Or, choose from a variety of complex carbohydrates like whole grains, vegetables, beans, baked potatoes, seeds and nuts. They are less harmful to blood sugar.

• • • •

FAULTY FAT
Separating the good from the bad

- Saturated fat is found in meats and whole dairy items. It can raise cholesterol, clogs arteries, and potentially promotes health woes like stroke, heart disease, obesity and even various cancers.

- Sources of healthy fats include: pure liquid vegetable oils (like olive oil and canola oil), fish oils, whole olives, nuts, avocado, flax seeds, and sunflower seeds. To avoid weight gain, use all fats in moderation, regardless of the source.

- Hydrogenated vegetable oils (a.k.a. trans fats) are also not recommended as they have been linked to heart disease and can raise cholesterol. They are commonly found in snack chips, salad dressings, mayonnaise, and peanut butter. Read food labels to avoid

- Make the switch to leaner meats like fish fillets and skinless poultry in place of red meat (beef and pork), opt for reduced-fat dairy items instead of whole.

· · · ·

FLAWED FLOUR

White flour is commonly used to make bread, pastry, cookies, crackers and noodles.

Most of the healthy nutrients which are naturally found in the kernel of whole grain wheat are processed out during the manufacture of white flour. These lost nutrients include the fiber, B-vitamins, vitamin E, and trace minerals.

- Don't be fooled by label advertising words like "enriched" as they only replace a modest portion of these nutrients, and these are often synthetics. Many breads and crackers may claim to be whole grain on the label, but if white flour is the first ingredient on the label there may only be a minor amount of whole grain added.
- Opt for "100% whole grain" instead. One way to check is to read the fiber content then compare the item to similar products. If a product has little or no fiber it may not contain much in the way of whole grain. Also, whole grain breads are usually heavier and darker in color than white bread.

· · · ·

STONEWALLING SALT

Sodium is an essential nutrient, but too much is linked to high blood pressure.

- Don't eliminate salt (sodium) entirely, just cut back! Most people get three to five times the amount that the human body requires.
- Read nutrition labels to avoid excess sodium added to commercially canned, boxed, and packaged foods.
- To help cut back, use herbs and seasoning blends to flavor foods at the dinner table.
- Natural sea salt is recommended over common table salt, offering less sodium and a higher ratio of favorable minerals.

FRIED FOODS

This includes common foods such as fried chicken, snack chips, French fries, onion rings, and deep-fried appetizers (like mushrooms and zucchini).

- Not only are these greasy foods excessively high in fat, but the type of oil used is often a hydrogenated version which has been known to raise cholesterol.
- Grill or roast your chicken instead of frying in oil. "Baked" snack chips (like pretzels) contain less oil than fried.

. . . .

CHOOSING COOKING FATS

The good, the bad, and the ugly.

Butter and lard are high in saturated fat which can contribute to heart disease. Many margarines may contain trans fats. So, if you desire to cut back on unhealthy fats, read the labels and compare selections with similar products.

- A good rule to remember is purchase the soft forms of butter or margarine which are sold in tubs rather than hard sticks. They are usually less saturated.
- Better yet, cook with pure liquid vegetable oil (such as olive). Vegetable oil sprays are also a good alternative.

. . . .

SUSPICIOUS SHELLFISH

Crab, lobster, clams, oysters, and shrimp.

Did you know that shellfish are scavengers of the sea? Basically, their function is cleaning up dead carcasses and other unhealthy debris lying on the ocean floor.

- Raw seafood (like oysters) can be full of bacteria that should be killed off by the heat of cooking. Many cases of food poisoning are linked to raw fish and shellfish consumption.

- Opt for fish fillets (fish with scales) instead.

• • • •

ARTIFICIAL SWEETENERS
The controversy lingers.

Perhaps these little packets of pink or blue are a better choice than fattening sugar which can be an important consideration to dieters and obese individuals.

However, they may be linked to various health woes because many of them are made up of chemicals. However, some have accused the sugar industry for making these accusations. Thus, the controversy lingers on just how good or bad they actually are.

The best advice is to use all sweeteners sparingly, regardless of the source.

• • • •

UTMOST UTENSILS
What you cook with can be just as important as what you eat.

- Much of the foods we microwave are commercially processed "quickie" meals; full of fats, salt, and chemicals. Additionally, "nuked" foods have most of their nutrients destroyed by the micro wave process leaving the consumer with nutritionally dead foods.
- For healthier alternatives to microwaving, steaming foods is actually best for veggies. Grill or roast meats.
- A hot air popcorn maker is the best bet for this snack. No oil is used in the cooking process and the popcorn comes out delicious.
- Cook with cast iron or stainless-steel cookware instead of aluminum, which is a toxic metal.

• • • •

NOTE: CONSULT YOUR PHYSICIAN FOR ALL QUESTIONS OR CONCERNS REGARDING THIS TOPIC OR ANY OTHER MATERIAL IN THIS BOOK.

• • • •

NOTE: NOT INTENDED TO PRESCRIBE OR DIAGNOSE. CONSULT YOUR PHYSICIAN FOR ALL HEALTH CONCERNS INCLUDING MEDICAL TREATMENTS, MEDICATIONS, DIETARY ALTERATIONS, VITAMIN SUPPLEMENTS, AND BEFORE STARTING A FITNESS PROGRAM.

FANTASTIC FIBER

Are you getting enough?

- A fiber-rich diet can help prevent ills such as diabetes, constipation, stroke, hypoglycemia, cancer, hemorrhoids, and obesity.
- Fiber is naturally abundant in most plant foods including vegetables, fruit, whole grains, and legumes (beans).
- Fiber is deficient in meats, dairy items, white flour, sugar, and salt.
- For optimum health adults need between 30 and 40 grams of fiber daily. Read nutrition labels ensure your diet contains adequate fiber.
- Fiber supplements are available in the form of psyllium, wheat bran, ground flax seed, and oat bran. They can be added to many foods such as pasta sauce, pizza, salads, eggs, sandwiches, casseroles, soups, rice dishes, cereals, baked goods, and more.

• • • •

OPT FOR OLIVE OIL

Mediterranean's are famed for using olive oil and their low rates of heart disease.

- It offers less saturated fat than other cooking fats like butter, lard, and gravy.
- Olive oil is recommended for all types of cooking needs.
- Oils aren't fat-free, so be sure to use in moderation if you are concerned about your weight.

• • • •

SUCCESSFUL SNACKING

- Go light on treats high in sugar, fat, or salt.
- Between meals eat more fruits and vegetables instead.
- Adopt nourishing snack habits. For example; plain popcorn, whole

grain crackers, raisins, prunes, carrot & celery sticks, low-fat yogurt, rice cakes, pretzels, baked chips, granola, dry-roasted nuts, natural peanut butter, bran muffins, sunflower seeds and whole grain cereals eaten as finger foods. (Be warned that many of these commercial snacks aren't calorie-free, so be sure to use in moderation!).

• • • •

CHOOSING CARBOHYDRATES

If you are going to eat carbs make sure you select the healthy types.

- Complex carbs burn slower and stabilize energy better than simple or refined white sugars.
- The good (recommended) carbs include whole grains such as oatmeal, brown rice, whole wheat, whole rye and whole barley. They also include whole fruits, vegetables, beans, peas, lentils, nuts, whole kernel corn, pumpkin, and sweet potatoes.
- The so-called 'white' carbs are not recommended. They include white sugar, white flour, white pasta, white rice, and white potatoes.
- Be warned that all carbs can potentially produce weight gain if not used in moderation.

• • • •

SPECIAL SPROUTS

- Healthy additions to sandwiches and salads, sprouts contain various vitamins, minerals and enzymes.
- They include alfalfa, broccoli, clover, sunflower, mustard, onion, lentil, radish, mung bean and soy.
- Sprouts should be consumed raw to preserve enzyme content.
- Be sure to refrigerate always to prevent spoilage.

• • • •

SUPERIOR SEA VEGETABLES

Since recorded history dried seaweeds have been utilized by cultures around the globe.

- They contain many valuable minerals essential to health, including iodine which prevents goiter.
- Renowned in Asia for use in soups, salads, and as sushi wrappers. Sold in U.S. health stores and Asian markets.

• • • •

HONORABLE HERBS and SPICES
Cut the fat, not the flavor in foods.

- As alternatives to high-fat sauces, dressings, and gravies try favoring your foods with various herbs and common kitchen spices.
- For eons, herbs have been popular worldwide as folk remedies and for enhancing food.
- Picking wild herbs on your own may pose health risks. Purchase thru a reputable dealer.

• • • •

DECADENT DESSERTS
Learn to save those sweet treats for special occasions only.

- For healthier desserts try whole fruits such as melons, apples, pears, oranges, grapes, berries, bananas, etc.
- Slice and mix various fruits together to create homemade fruit cocktail.
- Create healthy parfaits by layering low-fat yogurt with fruit in tall glasses, and serve chilled.

• • • •

GRAND GREEN TEA
On average, green tea drinkers outlive coffee drinkers.

- Popular beverage in China for centuries, and suspected of having life extension properties.

- Green teas are a superior source of anti-oxidants which are known to help prevent certain cancers and heart disease.
- Teas do not contain as much caffeine as coffee, but are not caffeine-free. Something to think about if you suffer from insomnia.

• • • •

FLEXIBLE FLAX SEEDS

- Flax seeds are packed with alpha-linolenic acid, the plant kingdom's version of Omega-3 fatty acids naturally found in fish oil.
- Flax seed oil may be just as effective as olive oil when it comes to protecting the heart and preventing breast cancer.

Try sprinkling some ground flax seed on breakfast cereal, tossed salads or stirring it into fruit juice, vegetable juice, soups, chili, and other prepared dishes.

• • • •

GREAT GARLIC & ONIONS
Known for their potent aromas and famous as a folk remedy.

- In various parts of the world, garlic and onions were common dietary staples of ancient civilizations.
- Hailed as miracle healers, capable of stimulating the immune system, slashing heart attack risk by preventing potentially fatal blood clots, preventing some types of cancer, and as effective antibiotics.
- They offer much flavor to foods, and an especially good time to cook with this potent pair is during cold and flu season, as researchers suggest they may offer preventive properties.

• • • •

BEVERAGE BLAST
There are good thirst quenchers along with the bad.

- **RECOMMENDED**: 100% fruit juice (no added sugars), vegetable juice, V-8 juice, bottled water, skim milk, green tea, herbal tea, and non-dairy milk made from soy, almond, or rice.

- **NOT RECOMMENDED**: drinks with added sugars such as soft drinks, sweetened juices, punches, custom coffees, whole dairy milk.

• • • •

CAGEY CONDIMENTS AND EXTRAS

Great for adding flavor to foods, but be cautious on your selections.

• LOW-FAT ITEMS INCLUDE: Mustard, salsa, relish, catsup, pickles, vinegar, vegetable broth, soy sauce, tomato sauce, herbs, spices, and vegetable oil sprays.

• HIGH-FAT CAUTIONS INCLUDE: Mayonnaise, creamy salad dressings, creamy dips, sour cream, meat gravy, lard, butter, margarine, and Alfredo sauce.

• • • •

NOTE: CONSULT YOUR PHYSICIAN FOR ALL QUESTIONS OR CONCERNS REGARDING THIS TOPIC OR ANY OTHER MATERIAL IN THIS BOOK.

• • • •

NOTE: NOT INTENDED TO PRESCRIBE OR DIAGNOSE. CONSULT YOUR PHYSICIAN FOR ALL HEALTH CONCERNS INCLUDING MEDICAL TREATMENTS, MEDICATIONS, DIETARY ALTERATIONS, VITAMIN SUPPLEMENTS, AND BEFORE STARTING A FITNESS PROGRAM.

HERBAL HOTSHOTS

Nature's incredible pharmacy.

• • • •

Dating back thousands of years and treasured by Romans, Chinese, Indians, Mayans, Incas, Aztecs & Egyptians; herbs are touted as remedies for all ailments and do-it-yourself cures. From Renaissance herbalists who recorded their information, to backwoods' cabin dwellers who simply passed down secrets through word-of-mouth to descendants, these natural remedies have much folklore in their long history.

- Herbal teas remain the most popular method of using herbs. Combinations are available featuring anywhere from 3 to 6 different herbs for specific uses, such as a "morning starter," "energizer blend," or a before bed "sleep-aid," etc. Check your health store or grocer for the many varieties.

• • • •

- Herb tea may be flavored with some natural honey and lemon juice, and can be a pleasant way of pursuing coffee substitution. Avoid adding refined sugar or cream to herb teas, especially if dieting.

• • • •

- If you buy "loose bulk" form instead of tea bags, it is recommended you purchase a handy device called "tea bells" or "tea spoons." These make them much easier to work with. They are perforated metal containers that prevent loose particles from wandering freely and requiring the use of strainers. Such gadgets sell in health stores at moderate prices.

Cautions and Disclaimer.

Remember that herbs are also medicines!

While some herbal teas are quite mild and may be used casually instead of coffee, others are very potent and should only be used sparingly for brief periods.

Some herbs may not mix well with other medications and may cause an allergic reaction.

Read labels for instructions.

Do not pick wild herbs for self-usage, but make your purchases through a health store.

Always know exactly what herbs you are taking and which effects to expect.

Consult your physician on all health matters, especially if ill or pregnant.

Contact a qualified herbalist for questions concerning specific applications of herbs.

• • • •

Herbs and Common Uses:

AGRIMONY.................. Stomach, diarrhea, kidneys, rheumatism.

ALFALFA..................... Arthritis, blood builder-purifier, ulcers.

ANGELICA.................. Headaches, coughs, colds, and stomach.

ANISE.......................... Stomach, tonic, stimulant, and nausea.

BAY............................. Indigestion, cramps, tonic and catarrh.

BEARBERRY................ Bladder, antiseptic, tonic and diuretic.

BIRCHLEAF................. Colds, fever, diuretic, boils, catarrh.

BUCHU....................... Diuretic, urinary, prostate and colon.

BUCKTHORN.............. Laxative, rheumatism, gout, dropsy.

BURDOCK................ Blood cleanser, swelling, hemorrhoids.

CATNIP.................... Insomnia, feverishness and convulsions.

CELERY SEED........... Nervous, liver, and gastric complaints.

CENTAURY................ Tonic, blood, exhaustion, and arthritis.

CHAMOMILE.............. Nerves, digestion, kidney, bronchial.

CAMPHOR.................. Gout, neuralgia, reproductive organs.

CHICORY.................. Tonic, laxative, diuretic, and kidneys.

CLEAVERS................ Kidney, bladder, urine, and also liver.

COMFREY................. Diarrhea, chest colds, and skin ulcer.

CORN SILK................ Bladder, urinary, rheumatic, kidney.

COUGH GRASS......... Colds, throat, fever, tonic and catarrh.

DANDELION............. Gastric, anemia, blood, gout and skin.

ELDER FLOWER....... Asthma, colds, influenza, and fever.

EUCALYPTUS............ Bronchial, coughs, colds and antiseptic.

EYEBRIGHT............... Vision, tonic, eyestrain and astringent.

FENNEL.................... Indigestion, arthritis, colon and colds.

FENUGREEK.............. Mucous, colds, fever, sinus, inflame.

GOLDEN ROD............ Digestion, kidney, colds, and cough.

GOLDEN SEAL........... All-purpose; from colds to nerves.

GROUND IVY............. Diarrhea, tonic, kidney and dyspepsia.

HOPS............................ Nerve, anemia, insomnia, appetite.

HOREHOUND.............. Cough, throat, stimulant, and tonic.

HUCKLEBERRY......... Digestive problems, and diarrhea.

HYSSOP....................... Nerve, fever, stomach, and purifier.

JUNIPER.................... Laxative, sinusitis, bladder, gonorrhea.

LAVENDER............... Nerve, sedative, tonic, nausea, stimulant.

LEMON TEA.............. Colds, tonic, fever, antiseptic and flu.

LOBELIA.................... Relaxant, heart, fever, coughs, lung.

LICORICE.................. Cough, throat, colitis and expectorant.

LINDEN..................... Indigestion, dyspepsia, mucous, nerve.

LUNGWORT.............. Lung, respiratory, influenza, chest.

MANDRAKE............... Cathartic, liver, bowels, and fever.

MANDRAKE ROOT.... Cathartic, nerve tonic, and insomnia.

MARIGOLD................ Tonic, heart, skin, and varicose vein.

MARJORAM............... Nerve, stomach, digest, and nausea.

MARSHMALLOW....... Colds, cough, throat, soreness, chest.

MINT.......................... Digestion, stomach, nerve, stimulant.

MISTLETOE............... Tonic, nerve, stimulant, and diuretic.

MULLEIN.................. Chest, hay fever, lung, warts, asthma.

NETTLE.................... Exhaustion, colon, blood and catarrh.

OAT......................... Nervousness, sleep, liver and lumbago.

OAT STRAW............. Muscles, insomnia, constipation, nerves.

ORANGE................... Carminative, stimulant, stomach, tonic.

PANSY...................... Heart, diuretic, laxative, jaundice, gout.

PAPAYA................... Digestion, indigestion, allergy, stomach.

PARSLEY................. Cleanser, glands, stomach and breath.

PLEURICE............... Diarrhea, dysentery, flu, rheumatism.

POKEWEED............ Rheumatic, anodyne, laxative, cathartic.

RASPBERRY............ Throat, nerves, menstrual and diarrhea.

RED CLOVER............ Used for all forms of tumors, cancer.

ROSE HIPS............... Colds, infusion, flu, stress and purifier.

ROSEMARY.............. Nerve, digestion, liver and migraine.

SAGE....................... Fever, constipation, nerve and throat.

SARSAPARILLA........... Cleanser, rheumatism, skin, urinary.

SASSAFRAS............. Skin, diarrhea, purifier, rheumatism.

SAW PALMETTO.... Endocrine, bronchial, colds and tonic.

SPRUCE................... Calmative, expectorant, diaphoretic.

SENNA.................... Laxative, cathartic, and vermifuge.

SHAVE GRASS......... Kidney, stomach, lung and diuretic.

SLIPPERY ELM........ Bronchial, mucous, bowels, diarrhea.

STRAWBERRY.......... Laxative, stomach, tonic and bowels.

THYME...................... Digestion, coughs, nerve and asthma.

UVA-URSI............... Diabetes, diuretic, kidney and bladder.

VALERIAN ROOT...... Nerve tonic, stimulant and insomnia.

WATERCRESS........... Diuretic, colds, gout and bloodstream.

YARROW.................. Pleurisy, pneumonia, ulcers and chest.

YELLOW DOCK........ Skin blemish, blood purifier, laxative.

YERBA SANTA......... Asthma, rheumatic, colds and bronchial.

· · · ·

Cautions and Disclaimer.

Remember that herbs are also medicines!

While some herbal teas are quite mild and may be used casually instead of coffee, others are very potent and should only be used sparingly for brief periods.

Some herbs may not mix well with other medications and may cause an allergic reaction.

Read labels for instructions.

Do not pick wild herbs for self-usage, but make your purchases through a health store.

Always know exactly what herbs you are taking and which effects to expect.

· · · ·

NOTE: CONSULT YOUR PHYSICIAN ON ALL HEALTH MATTERS, ESPECIALLY IF ILL, PREGNANT OR TAKING ANY MEDICATION.

· · · ·

CONSULT YOUR PHYSICIAN FOR ALL QUESTIONS OR CONCERNS REGARDING HERBS OR ANY OTHER MATERIAL IN THIS BOOK.

• • • •

YOU MAY WISH TO CONTACT A QUALIFIED HERBALIST FOR QUESTIONS CONCERNING SPECIFIC APPLICATIONS OF HERBS.

• • • •

• VARIOUS CONDITIONS AND HERBS

ACNE
Valerian, strawberry, angelica, chamomile.

• • • •

ANTI-DEPRESSIVE
Gotu kola, kelp, ginseng, capsium, yarrow, ergot.

• • • •

ANEMIA
Alfalfa, chive, artichoke, dandelion, comfrey, beet.

• • • •

ADRENAL
Ginger, gotu kola, mullein, hawthorn, ginseng, cayenne.

• • • •

ALLERGIES Golden seal, chaparral, parsley, burdock, lobelia, brigham, marshmallow.

• • • •

ARTHRITIS & RHEUMATISM

Yucca, sarsaparilla, alfalfa, burdock.

. . . .

ARTERIOSCLEROSIS
Alfalfa, black elder, burdock, comfrey.

. . . .

ASTHMA
Pleurisy root, muellin, blessed thistle horehound.

. . . .

BACKACHES
Arnica, vervain, black cohosh, juniper, betony.

. . . .

BAD BREATH
Caraway, dill, myrrh, parsley.

. . . .

BED WETTING
Lemon, fennel seed, pansy, yarrow.

. . . .

BLOOD PURIFIER
Echinacea, red clover, golden seal, dandelion.

. . . .

BONE PROBLEMS Alfalfa, horsetail, oat, comfrey.

. . . .

BRUISES
Aloe vera, comfrey, fenugreek, calendula.

. . . .

BURNS

Aloe vera, comfrey, olive, calendula.

• • • •

BLOOD PRESSURE (High or low)

Cayenne, garlic, kelp, ginger, parsley, golden seal, ginseng.

• • • •

CALCIUM DEFICIENCY

Horsetail, comfrey, oat straw, lobelia, alfalfa.

• • • •

CANCER

Red clover, garlic, burdock, pau d'arco.

• • • •

CLEANSER

Rhubarb, cascara sagrada, ginger.

• • • •

COLITIS

Ginger, comfrey, marshmallow.

• • • •

COLDS (and flu)

Rose hips, garlic, golden seal, cayenne.

• • • •

DIGESTION

Comfrey, cayenne, Irish moss, golden seal.

• • • •

DIABETES

Dandelion, fenugreek, golden seal, kelp.

. . . .

DIZZINESS
Catnip, Hawthorne, lemon, peppermint.

. . . .

EMPHYSEMA
Lungwort, celery, elderberry, plantain.

. . . .

FEVER
Catnip, arnica, thyme, blue vervain, fenugreek.

. . . .

FEMALE HORMONE
Golden seal, raspberry, marshmallow, licorice.

. . . .

GARGLE
Peppermint, comfrey, chamomile, parsley.

. . . .

GASTRO-INTESTINAL
Golden seal, comfrey, cayenne, slippery elm.

. . . .

GALLSTONES
Barberry, vervain, aloe vera, alder, dandelion.

. . . .

GENERAL TONIC
Golden seal, licorice, comfrey, ginseng, kelp.

GLAND PROBLEMS

Comfrey, mullein, lobelia, black walnut.

• • • •

GOUT

Cranberry, burdock, birch, celery, arnica.

• • • •

HAY FEVER

Black cohosh, skullcap, pleurisy, cubeb, papaya.

• • • •

HEALER (general)

Comfrey, rose hips, aloe, kelp, alfalfa.

• • • •

HEART

Cayenne, kelp, arnica, hawthorn, wood betany.

• • • •

HEMORRHOIDS

Chamomile, nettle, aloe.

• • • •

HYPOGLYCEMIA

Licorice, dandelion, horseradish, safflower.

• • • •

IMPOTENCE

Ginseng, saw palmetto, fo-ti, gotu kola, kelp.

• • • •

INSOMNIA
Skullcap, valerian, hops, chamomile.

• • • •

INFECTION (general)
Garlic, comfrey, blue vervain, chinchona.

• • • •

IRON
Beet powder, yellow dock, nettle, burdock.

• • • •

KIDNEY
Cranberry, parsley, uva ursi, dandelion.

• • • •

LACTATION
Basil, borage, anise, dill, nettle, alfalfa.

• • • •

LAXATIVES
Senna, buckthorn, anise, licorice, alfalfa, fennel.

• • • •

LIVER PROBLEMS
Dandelion, licorice, beet, oat, rhubarb, cranberry.

• • • •

LUNG & CHEST
Mullein, marshmallow, pleurisy, comfrey.

• • • •

MALE HORMONE

Ginseng, gotu kola, echinacea, damiana.

· · · ·

MEMORY
Gotu kola, cayenne, blessed thistle, ginger.

· · · ·

MENOPAUSE
Black cohosh, licorice, ginseng, squawvine.

· · · ·

NERVOUSNESS
Black cohosh, valerian, thyme, capsium, ginger.

· · · ·

PAIN
Wood betany, raspberry, rosemary, saw palmetto.

· · · ·

PANCREAS
Uvi ursi, licorice, mullein, cayenne, golden seal.

· · · ·

PARASITES
Garlic, male fern, tansy, black walnut, comfrey.

· · · ·

PRE-NATAL
Black cohosh, alfalfa, penny royal, raspberry.

· · · ·

PROSTATE
Parsley, saw palmetto, buchu, uvi ursi, kelp.

· · · ·

PURIFIER
Chaparral, alfalfa, kelp, aloe vera, golden seal.

· · · ·

RESPIRATORY
Marshmallow, mullein, comfrey, chickweed.

· · · ·

SKIN
Dandelion, alfalfa, kelp, parsley, chickweed.

· · · ·

SINUS
Cayenne, golden seal, burdock, marshmallow.

· · · ·

TEETH AND GUMS
Horsetail, white oak, clove, balm, oat straw, comfrey.

· · · ·

THYROID
Kelp, black walnut, Irish moss, cayenne.

· · · ·

ULCERS
Myrrh, golden seal, cayenne, garlic.

· · · ·

VARICOSE VEIN
Rose hips, sassafras, arnica, hawthorn.

· · · ·

WEIGHT CONTROL

Kelp, saffron, chickweed, celery, burdock, papaya.

. . . .

Cautions and Disclaimer.

Remember that herbs are also medicines!

While some herbal teas are quite mild and may be used casually instead of coffee, others are very potent and should only be used sparingly for brief periods.

Some herbs may not mix well with other medications and may cause an allergic reaction.

Read labels for instructions.

Do not pick wild herbs for self-usage, but make your purchases through a health store.

Always know exactly what herbs you are taking and which effects to expect.

. . . .

NOTE: CONSULT YOUR PHYSICIAN ON ALL HEALTH MATTERS, ESPECIALLY IF ILL, PREGNANT OR TAKING ANY MEDICATION.

. . . .

CONSULT YOUR PHYSICIAN FOR ALL QUESTIONS OR CONCERNS REGARDING HERBS OR ANY OTHER MATERIAL IN THIS BOOK.

. . . .

NOTE: NOT INTENDED TO PRESCRIBE OR DIAGNOSE. CONSULT YOUR PHYSICIAN FOR ALL HEALTH CONCERNS INCLUDING MEDICAL TREATMENTS, MEDICATIONS, DIETARY ALTERATIONS, VITAMIN SUPPLEMENTS, AND BEFORE STARTING A FITNESS PROGRAM.

. . . .

YOU MAY WISH TO CONTACT A QUALIFIED HERBALIST FOR
QUESTIONS CONCERNING SPECIFIC APPLICATIONS OF
HERBS.

• • • •

*"Doctors are men who prescribe medicines of which they know little, to cure
diseases of which they know less, in human beings of whom they know
nothing." -Voltaire*

Confused? These tips may help:

• • • •

- 3 ounces chicken or fish = Deck of cards
- 1 cup of vegetables = Size of your fist
- Medium apple = Size of a baseball
- Half cup pasta, cooked = Ice cream scoop
- and 1/2-ounces cheese = Pair of dominoes
- 1 teaspoon butter/margarine = Tip of your thumb
- 1 cup dry cereal = Large handful

BIBLICAL WELL-BEING

Medicine for Your Soul.

• • • •

"God heals and the doctor takes the fee." -Ben Franklin

• • • •

"Feed your faith and starve your doubts to death." -Pastor Lester Sumrall

• • • •

Where to look in the Bible.

• • • •

The Holy Bible is loaded with passages about sickness and health. The key to unlocking God's grace is to read it every day, believe in what you have read, and make prayer part of your daily ritual. You will also find that God works in mysterious ways.

• • • •

In regards to faith healing some people are healed rather quickly, while others are led in a particular direction required for healing over time.

• • • •

Some are not healed at all. What we must realize is that when we do our part God does his. He'll meet us halfway. In other words, by taking better care of ourselves thru proper diet, exercise, etc. we please God and open ourselves up to his blessings.

• • • •

You are what you eat, and remember to treat your body with respect like the temple he has created within us.

† IS ANY AMONG YOU AFFLICTED?
Read James 5: 13-15.
† WHEN IN SICKNESS
Read Psalm 41.
† FOR REST & PEACE
Read Matthew 11:25-30.
† WHEN DISCOURAGED
Read Psalm 34.
† TO KNOW GOD'S WILL FOR YOUR LIFE
Read Proverbs 3:1-6.
† WHEN YOU NEED COURAGE
Read Joshua 1:1-9.
† WHEN YOU NEED ASSURANCE
Read Romans 8.
† GUIDELINES FOR LIVING
Read Matthew 5-7; Romans 12.

• • • •

BELOW ARE SOME OF THE HEALTH-RELATED VERSES FOUND IN THE BIBLE:

† *"Feed me, I pray thee, with that same red pottage, for I am faint. Then Jacob gave Esau bread and pottage of lentils, and he did eat and drink and went his way." Genesis 25:29-34*

† *"Take thou also unto thee wheat and barley, and beans, and lentils and millet, and fiches, and put them into one vessel, and make thee bread thereof." Ezekiel 4:9*

† *"It is good not to eat meat or to drink wine, or to do anything by which your brother stumbles." Romans 14:21*

† *"He said, 'If you listen carefully to the voice of the Lord your God and do what is right in His eyes, if you pay attention to His commands and keep all of His decrees, I will not bring on you any of the diseases I brought on the Egyptians, for I am the Lord, who heals you.' " Exodus 15:26*

† *"And the Lord will take away from thee all sickness..." Deuteronomy 7:15*

† *"...by His wounds you have been healed." 1 Peter 2:24*

† *"He helps the brokenhearted and binds their wounds." Psalms 147:3*

† *"Even though I walk through the valley of the shadow of death, I will fear no evil, for you are with me; your rod and your staff, they comfort me." Psalms 23:4*

† *"Bless the Lord, O my soul, and forget none of His benefits; Who pardons all your iniquities; Who heals all your diseases; Who redeems your life from the pit; Who crowns you with loving kindness and compassion; Who satisfies your years with good things, So that your youth is renewed like an eagle." Psalms 103:1-5*

† *"Praise the Lord, my soul, and never forget all the good he has done: He is the one who forgives all your sins, the one who heals all your diseases." Psalms 103:2-3*

† *"Do not be wise in your own eyes; fear and respect the Lord and shun evil. This will bring health to your body and nourishment to your bones." Proverbs 3:7-8*

† *"Above all else, guard your heart, for it is the wellspring of life." Proverbs 4:23*

† *"Hope deferred makes the heart sick; but when hopes are realized at last, there is life and joy." Proverbs 13:12*

† "A heart at peace gives life to the body, but envy rots the bones." *Proverbs 14:30*

† "When a man is gloomy, everything seems to go wrong; when he is cheerful (and full of hope), everything seems right." *Proverbs 15:15*

† "A cheerful heart is good medicine." *Proverbs 17:22*

† "A man's spirit can sustain his broken body, but when spirit dies, what hope is left?" *Proverbs 18:14*

† "Know that wisdom is sweet to your soul; if you find it, there is hope and it will not be cut off." *Proverbs 24:14*

† "They will turn to the Lord, and He will respond to their pleas and heal them." *Isaiah 19:22*

† Surely, He (God) hath borne our sicknesses [kholee, infirmities], and carried our sorrows [makob, pains, diseases]. *Isaiah 53:4*

† "I have carried you since you were born; I have taken care of you from your birth. Even when you are old, I will be the same. Even when your hair has turned gray, I will take care of you. I will sustain you and I will rescue you." *Isaiah 46:3-4*

† 'He gives strength to the weary and increases the power of the weak. Even youths grow tired and weary, and young men stumble and fall; but those who hope in the Lord will renew their strength. They will soar on wings like an eagle; they will run and not grow weary; they will walk and not faint'. *Isaiah 40:28-31*

† "Why spend money on what is not bread, and your labor on what does not satisfy? Listen, listen to Me and eat what is good, and your soul will delight in the richest of fare." *Isaiah 55:2*

† *"The Lord will guide you always; He will satisfy your needs... and will strengthen your frame. You will be like a well-watered garden, like a spring whose waters never fail." Isaiah 58:11*

† *"This is what the Lord says, 'Your wound is incurable, your injury is beyond healing. There is no one to plead your cause, no remedy for your sore, no healing for you. All your allies have forgotten you; they care nothing for you. ... But I will restore you to health and heal your wounds...'" Jeremiah 30:12-14, 17*

† *"My People are destroyed from lack of knowledge". Hosea 4:6*

† *"You cannot add any time to your life by worrying about it." Matthew 6:27*

† *"So, don't be anxious about tomorrow. God will take care of your tomorrow too. Live one day at a time." Matthew 6:34*

† *When evening came, many who were demon-possessed were brought to HIM and He drove out the spirits with His word and healed all that were sick. This was to fulfill what was spoken through the prophet Isaiah: "He took up our infirmities and carried our diseases." Matthew 8:16-17*

† *"Jesus... said, "With man this is impossible, but with God all things are possible." Matthew 19:26*

† *"...if you can do anything ...help us." "If you can?" said Jesus. "Everything is possible for HIM who believes." Mark 9:23*

† *"Jesus said unto them, 'Surely you will quote this proverb to Me: Physician, heal yourself.'" Luke 4:23*

† *"Your faith has healed you. Go in peace." Luke 8:48*

† *"And take heed to yourselves, lest at any time your hearts be overcharged with surfeiting (overeating), and drunkenness, and cares of this life, and so that day come upon you unawares." Luke 21:34*

† *"Peace I leave with you; my peace I give you. I do not give to you as the world gives. Do not let your hearts be troubled and do not be afraid." John 14:27*

† *"If you abide in Me and My Word abides in you, ask what you will and it shall be done unto you." John 15:7*

† *"...how God anointed Jesus of Nazareth with the Holy Spirit and power, and how he went around doing good and healing all who were under the power of the devil, because god was with HIM. Acts 10:38*

† *"But we... rejoice in our sufferings, because we know that suffering produces perseverance; perseverance, character; and character, hope." Romans 3:5*

† *"May the God of hope fill you with all joy and peace as you trust in HIM, so that you may overflow with hope by the power of the Holy Spirit." Romans 15:13*

† *"You were bought at a price [Jesus death on the cross]. Therefore, honor God with your body. 1 Corinthians 6:20*

† *"The things we see now (including illness and suffering) are here today, gone tomorrow. But the things we cannot see now will last forever." 1 Corinthians 7:31.*

† *"God keeps His promise, and He will not allow you to be tested beyond your power to remain firm; at the time you are put to the test, He will give you strength to endure it, and so provide you with a way out." 1 Corinthians 10:13*

† *But thanks be to God, who in Christ always leads us in triumph, and through us spreads the fragrance of the knowledge of HIM everywhere."* 2 Corinthians 2:14

† *"Do not be anxious about anything, but in everything, by prayer and petition, with Thanksgiving, present your requests to God. And the peace of God, which transcends all understanding, will guard your hearts and your minds in Christ Jesus."* Philippians 4:6

† *"I can do all things through Christ who strengthens me."* Philippians 4:13

† *"...I pray that you may enjoy good health and that all may go well with you, even as your soul is getting along well."* 3 John 1:2

• • • •

NOTE: Information presented throughout this book is not intended to prescribe or diagnose. Consult your physician for all health concerns.

AUTHOR PROFILE

With more than twenty years' experience as a nutritional researcher and author A.J. Fleming, N.D. was a naturopathic consultant, former adviser to a vitamin supplement manufacturer, magazine contributor, newspaper columnist, and personal health counselor. An ex-marathon runner with the Boston Marathon to his credit, his hobbies include reading, fitness, and vegan cooking.

Books by A.J. Fleming, N.D.

THE NATURAL WAY.
STOP Committing Suicide with a Fork!

• • • •

Did You Know That 3 Out Of 4 Ailments Are Preventable?
That's an amazing seventy-five percent! If less pain, fewer trips to the doctor, lower medical bills, fewer medications and less surgery in favor of alternative medicine sound appealing, then this program is for you. Learn the natural health secrets that can help trim that waistline, help you look and feel better, increase energy, and live longer!

• • • •

Prevent or reverse common ills such as high blood pressure, heart disease, diabetes, cancer, arthritis, stroke, constipation, insomnia, osteoporosis, migraines, chronic fatigue, and more. A complete health program featuring valuable tips on prevention, life extension, fitness, health foods, nutrients, supplements, fiber, herbs, vegetarianism, food combining, juice fasting, and more!

• • • •

Here you will discover all the natural health secrets that evolved from the famed quote, "You are what you eat!" Includes vegetarian-friendly food tips, plus Bible health quotes for spiritual enrichment. Learn the secrets of preventing and overcoming ailments the natural way.

• • • •

A Must For Any Health Library!

• • • •

To Order: www.healselfnaturally.weebly.com

Nutrition Made E-Z

• • • •

Health care and skyrocketing medical costs in the U.S. has reached an all-time crisis. America is the richest nation in the world but also boasts the highest rates of cancer, heart disease, and obesity. Far too many adults and children alike are grossly overweight.

• • • •

Many of this nation's health woes are caused by a deluge of popular and readily available foods that are overloaded with fat, sugar, and salt while simultaneously lacking in essential nutrients such as vitamins, minerals, antioxidants, phytonutrients and fiber. Additionally, a sedentary lifestyle from our obsession with electronics like computers, cable and satellite television, and video games escalates the obesity problem.

• • • •

In this book you will learn how to convert favorite junk foods into healthy meals, plus all you need to know about the basics of eating right for optimum health. If you are confused about nutrition this book offers quick facts at a glance, information on nutrients, healthy foods, do's and don'ts, fitness tips and more. It is designed to offer helpful hints that can prevent ills, shed pounds, make you look better, feel better, and live a longer, healthier & happier life! Designed for simple study.

• • • •

Learn the general basics of nutrition in a weekend. Includes vegetarian-friendly eating tips, herbal medicine and biblical health passages (medicine for your soul). Educational joy for the entire family. Intended for ages 9 to 99.

• • • •

Hopefully, this book will make a difference and help educate people on the fundamentals of a fit lifestyle, and better eating habits for improved health. Good luck and may God bless all those who seek better health.

www.ingramcontent.com/pod-product-compliance
Lightning Source LLC
Chambersburg PA
CBHW070433290526
45791CB00005B/1949